Super]

Plant Based Diet Cookbook

Amazingly Delicious Recipes to Lose
Weight, Balance Hormones, Boost
Brain Health, and Reverse Disease

Margaret Burton

TABLE OF CONTENTS

INTRODUCTION

There are several debates about which diet is the most beneficial to your health. Despite this, many health and wellness communities will agree that diets that prioritize organic and whole ingredients while limiting refined foods are the best for overall wellness. And, as you would expect, the plant-based whole foods diet would excel at this. Let's take a look at how this diet works and what this type of eating is all about so you can apply it to your own needs.

There is no specific description of what this type of diet entails because it is all about eating well and ensuring that our bodies get all of the nutrients they need from plant sources. Since there are different plant-based diets to choose from, each one can differ depending on how much an individual chooses to include or remove animal products from their diet. Some vegetarians, for example, eat fish, while others are vegan and do not consume any animal products.

It is a common reality that the best way to have the greatest effect on our weight is to keep track of what we eat. A plant-based diet allows you to enjoy automatic, quick fat burning without the calorie restrictions that other diets impose.

Weight loss is almost a foregone conclusion once you begin a plant-based diet, but it is far from the only advantage you can experience. Consider all of the things you've always wanted to do but have put off because you just don't have the stamina after a long day at work.

Now is the best time to dust off those hobbies and pastimes, because eating a plant-based diet will give you more energy for your everyday work and play! The diet's resulting mental insight and sharpness of thinking are also beneficial results. A better health report card, in the form of optimized cholesterol readings, normalized blood sugar, and a correspondingly reduced risk of cardiovascular disorders, are only a few of the health benefits that most people on the diet encounter.

BREAKFAST RECIPES

1. Chocolate Chip Banana Pancake

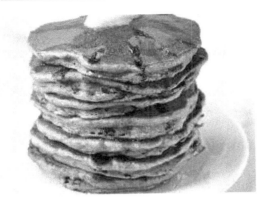

Preparation Time: 15 minutes

Cooking Time: 3 minutes

Servings: 6

Ingredients:

- 1 large ripe banana, mashed
- 2 tablespoons coconut sugar
- 3 tablespoons coconut oil, melted
- 1 cup of coconut milk
- 1 ½ cups whole wheat flour
- 1 teaspoon baking soda
- ½ cup vegan chocolate chips
- Olive oil, for frying

Directions:

1. Grab a large bowl and add the banana, sugar, oil, and milk. Stir well. Add the flour and baking soda and stir again until combined.

2. Add the chocolate chips and fold through, then pop to one side. Put a skillet over medium heat and add a drop of oil.

3. Pour ¼ of the batter into the pan and move the pan to cover. Cook for 3 minutes, then flip and cook on the other side. Repeat with the remaining pancakes, then serve and enjoy.

Nutrition: Calories: 105 Fat: 13g Carbs: 23g Protein: 5g

2. Avocado and 'Sausage' Breakfast Sandwich

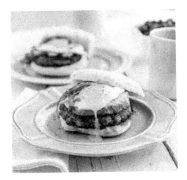

Preparation Time: 15 minutes

Cooking Time: 10 minutes

Servings: 1

Ingredients:

- 1 vegan sausage patty
- 1 cup kale, chopped
- 2 teaspoons extra virgin olive oil
- 1 tablespoon pepitas
- Salt and pepper, to taste
- 1 tablespoon vegan mayo
- 1/8 teaspoon chipotle powder
- 1 teaspoon jalapeno chopped
- 1 English muffin, toasted
- ¼ avocado, sliced

Directions:

1. Place a sauté pan over high heat and add a drop of oil. Add the vegan patty and cook for 2 minutes. Flip the patty, then add the kale and pepitas.

2. Season well, then cook for another few minutes until the patty is cooked. Find a small bowl and add the mayo, chipotle powder, and jalapeno. Stir well to combine.

3. Place the muffin onto a flat surface, spread with the spicy mayo, then top with the patty. Add the sliced avocado, then serve and enjoy.

Nutrition: Calories: 573 Fat: 23g Carbs: 36g Protein: 21g

3. Cinnamon Rolls with Cashew Frosting

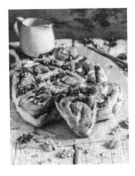

Preparation Time: 25 minutes

Cooking Time: 25 minutes

Servings: 12

Ingredients:

- 3 tablespoons vegan butter
- ¾ cup unsweetened almond milk
- ½ teaspoon salt
- 3 tablespoons caster sugar
- 1 teaspoon vanilla extract
- ½ cup pumpkin puree
- 3 cups all-purpose flour
- 2 ¼ teaspoons dried active yeast
- 3 tablespoons softened vegan butter
- 3 tablespoons brown sugar
- ½ teaspoon cinnamon

- ½ cup cashews

- ½ cup icing sugar

- 1 teaspoon vanilla extract

- 2/3 cup almond milk

Directions:

1. Soak the cashews for 1 hour in boiling water. Grease a baking sheet and pop to one side. Find a small bowl, add the butter, and pop into the microwave to melt.

2. Add the sugar and stir well, then set aside to cool. Grab a large bowl and add the flour, salt, and yeast. Stir well to mix.

3. Place the cooled butter into a jug, add the pumpkin puree, vanilla, and almond milk. Stir well together. Pour the wet fixings into the dry and stir well to combine.

4. Tip onto a flat surface and knead for 5 minutes, adding extra flour as needed to avoid sticking. Pop back into the bowl, cover with plastic wrap and pop into the fridge overnight.

5. Remove the dough from the fridge and punch down with your fingers. Using a rolling pin, roll to form an 18" rectangle, then spread with butter.

6. Find a small bowl and add the sugar and cinnamon. Mix well, then sprinkle with the butter. Roll the dough into a large sausage, then slice into sections.

7. Place onto the greased baking sheet and leave in a dark place to rise for one hour—Preheat the oven to 350°F. Strain the cashews and put them in your blender. Whizz until smooth.

8. Add the sugar and the vanilla, then whizz again. Add the almond milk until it reaches your desired consistency.

9. Pop into the oven and bake for 20 minutes until golden. Pour the glaze over the top, then serve and enjoy.

Nutrition: Calories: 243 Fat: 9g Carbs: 34g Protein: 4g

4. Vegan Variety Poppy Seed Scones

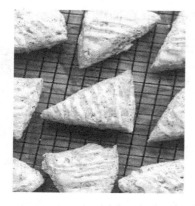

Preparation Time: 5 minutes

Cooking Time: 10 minutes

Servings: 12.

Ingredients:

- 1 cup white sugar
- 2 cups flour
- Juice from 1 lemon
- Zest from 1 lemon
- 4 teaspoon baking powder
- ½ teaspoon salt
- 1 cup Earth Balance or vegan butter
- 2 tablespoon poppy seeds
- ½ cup soymilk
- 1/3 cup water

Directions:

1. Warm oven to 400°F. Next, mix the sugar, the flour, the powder, and the salt in a big mixing bowl.

2. Add the vegan butter to the mixture and cut it up until you create a sand-like mixture. Next, add the lemon juice, the lemon zest, and the poppy seeds. Add the water and the soy milk, and stir the ingredients well.

3. Portion the batter out over a baking sheet in about ¼ cup portions. Allow the scones to bake for fifteen minutes and let them cool before serving. Enjoy.

Nutrition: Calories: 205 Fat: 3g Carbs: 12g Protein: 6g

5. Sweet Pomegranate Porridge

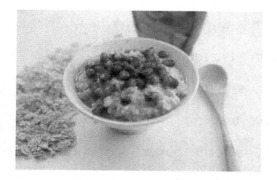

Preparation Time: 5 minutes

Cooking Time: 20 minutes

Servings: 4

Ingredients:

- 2 cups oats
- 1 ½ cups water
- 1 ½ cups pomegranate juice
- 2 tablespoons Pomegranate Molasses

Directions:

1. Pour all fixings into the instant pot and mix well. Seal the lid, and cook on high pressure for four minutes. Use a quick release, and serve warm.

Nutrition: Calories: 177 Fat: 6g Carbs: 23g Protein: 8g

6. <u>Apple Oatmeal</u>

Preparation Time: 5 minutes

Cooking Time: 20 minutes

Servings: 4

Ingredients:

- ¼ teaspoon of sea salt
- 1 cup cashew milk
- 1 cup strawberries, halved & fresh
- 1 tablespoon brown sugar
- 2 cups apples, diced
- 3 cups of water
- ¼ teaspoon coconut oil
- ½ cup steel cut oats

Directions:

1. Start by greasing your instant pot with oil, and add everything to it except for the milk and berries.
2. Cook on high pressure within ten minutes. Then add in your milk and strawberries after a natural pressure release. Mix well, and serve warm.

Nutrition: Calories: 435 Fat: 7g Carbs: 34g Protein: 8g

7. Breakfast Cookies

Preparation Time: 10 minutes

Cooking Time: 6 minutes

Servings: 24-32

Ingredients:

Dry Ingredients:

- ½ teaspoon baking powder
- 2 cups rolled oats
- ½ teaspoon baking soda

Wet Ingredients:

- 1 teaspoon pure vanilla extract
- 2 flax eggs (2 tbsp ground flaxseed & around 6 tablespoons of water, mix and put aside for 15 minutes)
- 2 tablespoons melted coconut oil
- 2 tablespoons pure maple syrup
- ½ cup natural creamy peanut butter
- 2 ripe bananas

Add-in Ingredients:

- ½ cup finely chopped walnuts
- ½ cup raisins

Optional Topping:

- 2 tablespoons chopped walnuts
- 2 tablespoons raisins

Directions:

1. Warm oven to 325°F, use parchment paper to line a baking sheet, and put it aside.
2. Put the bananas to a large bowl, and then use a fork to mash them until smooth. Add in the other wet ingredients and mix until well incorporated.
3. Add the dry ingredients and then use a rubber spatula to stir and fold them into the dry ingredients until well mixed. Stir in the walnuts and raisins.
4. Spoon the cookie dough onto your prepared baking sheet, ensuring that you leave adequate space between the cookies.
5. Bake in the preheated oven for around 12 minutes. Once ready, let the cookies cool on the baking sheet for around 10 minutes.
6. Lift the cookies carefully from the baking sheet onto a cooling rack to further cool.

Nutrition: Calories: 565 Fat: 6g Carbs: 32g Protein: 8g

8. Vegan Breakfast Biscuits

Preparation Time: 10 minutes

Cooking Time: 10 min

Servings: 6

Ingredients:

- 2 cups Almond Flour
- 1 tbsp Baking Powder
- ¼ teaspoon Salt
- ½ teaspoon Onion Powder
- ½ cup Coconut Milk
- ¼ cup Nutritional Yeast
- 2 tbsp Ground Flax Seeds
- ¼ cup Olive Oil

Directions:

1. Preheat oven to 450°F. Whisk together all ingredients in a bowl. Divide the batter into a pre-greased muffin tin. Bake for 10 minutes.

Nutrition: Calories: 432 Fat: 5g Carbs: 13g Protein: 8g

9. Orange French Toast

Preparation Time: 5 minutes

Cooking Time: 30 minutes

Servings: 8 servings

Ingredients:

- 2 cups of plant milk (unflavored)
- 4 tablespoon maple syrup
- 11/2 tablespoon cinnamon
- Salt (optional)
- 1 cup flour (almond)
- 1 tablespoon orange zest
- 8 bread slices

Directions:

1. Turn the oven and heat to 400°F afterward. In a cup, add ingredients and whisk until the batter is smooth.
2. Dip each piece of bread into the paste and permit to soak for a couple of seconds. Put in the pan, and cook until lightly browned.
3. Put the toast on the cookie sheet and bake for ten to fifteen minutes in the oven until it is crispy.

Nutrition: Calories: 129 Fat: 1.1g Carbs: 21.5g Protein: 7.9g

10. Chocolate Chip Coconut Pancakes

Preparation Time: 5 minutes

Cooking Time: 30 minutes

Servings: 8 servings

Ingredients:

- 11/4 cup oats
- 2 teaspoons coconut flakes
- 2 cup plant milk
- 11/4 cup maple syrup
- 11/3 cup of chocolate chips
- 2 1/4 cups buckwheat flour
- 2 teaspoon baking powder
- 1 teaspoon vanilla essence
- 2 teaspoon flaxseed meal
- Salt (optional)

Directions:

1. Put the flaxseed and cook over medium heat until the paste becomes a little moist. Remove seeds. Stir the buckwheat, oats, coconut chips, baking powder, and salt with each other in a wide dish.

2. In a large dish, stir together the retained flax water with the sugar, maple syrup, vanilla essence. Transfer the wet fixings to the dry ingredients and shake to combine.

3. Place over medium heat the nonstick grill pan. Pour 1/4 cup flour onto the grill pan with each pancake, and scatter gently. Cook for five to six minutes before the pancakes appear somewhat crispy.

Nutrition: Calories: 198 Fat: 9.1g Carbs: 11.5g Protein: 7.9g

LUNCH

11. Shio Koji Karaage Tofu

Preparation time: 15 minutes

Cooking time: 10 minutes

Servings: 4

Ingredients:

- Extra light olive oil (for deep-frying)
- 1 12-oz. pack extra firm tofu (drained, cubed)
- 4 tbsp. Hikari Shio Koji
- 1 tsp. fresh ginger (finely chopped)
- 1 garlic clove (minced)
- 2 tsp. soy sauce
- ½ cup almond flour
- Optional: lemon wedges

Directions:

1. Combine the tofu cubes with the Hikari Shio Koji, ginger, garlic, and soy sauce in a large bowl or Ziploc bag.

2. Use your hands to make sure the tofu is evenly coated. Cover the bowl or close the Ziploc bag and put it in the fridge. Marinate the tofu for at least 30 minutes up to a maximum of 1 day.

3. Heat a pot with enough olive oil to deep fry the tofu cubes. The ideal temperature for the oil is 325°F /160°F.

4. Take the tofu cubes out of the fridge and cover the cubes with almond flour. It can be done in a bowl or Ziploc bag. Use your hands to coat all tofu cubes with flour evenly.

5. Drop the coated cubes gently into the pot and fry until they're lightly browned. When the tofu cubes are ready, transfer them to a plate lined with paper towels to drain the excess oil.

6. Serve the shio koji karaage tofu, garnished with the optional lemon wedges if desired, and enjoy!

Nutrition: Calories: 355 Carbs: 4.9 g. Fat: 32 g. Protein: 11.3 g.

12. Zoodle Pesto Salad

Preparation time: 15 minutes

Cooking time: 0 minutes

Servings: 2

Ingredients:

- 2 medium zucchinis (spiralized into zoodles or sliced lengthwise very thinly)
- ¼ cup extra virgin olive oil
- 1 ½ cups fresh baby spinach leaves
- ¼ cup walnuts (crushed)
- 1 tsp. garlic powder
- Sea salt and ground black pepper to taste
- ¼ cup capers (chopped)
- Optional: ½ cup of vegan cheese

Directions:

1. Combine all the ingredients except the zoodles, capers, and optional vegan cheese in a food processor or blender. Pulse for 1-2 minutes into a smooth pesto.
2. If desired, cook zoodles or zucchini slices for up to 4 minutes in a large skillet, boiling water, and a pinch of

olive oil over medium heat. Alternatively, the zoodles or zucchini slices can be used raw.

3. Melt the optional vegan cheese on a plate in the microwave for about 40 seconds until it is melted and spreadable.

4. Serve the raw or cooked zoodles with the pesto, garnished with the chopped capers. Top the dish with the optional molten vegan cheese and add more salt and pepper to taste. Serve and enjoy!

Nutrition: Calories: 389 Carbs: 6.5 g. Fat: 37 g. Protein: 5.9 g.

13. Cucumber Edamame Salad

Preparation time: 45 minutes

Cooking time: 10 minutes

Servings: 2

Ingredients:

- 3 tbsp. avocado oil
- 1 cup cucumber (sliced into thin rounds)
- ½ cup fresh sugar snap peas (sliced or whole)
- ½ cup fresh edamame
- ¼ cup radish (sliced)
- 1 large Hass avocado (peeled, pitted, sliced)
- 1 nori sheet (crumbled)
- 2 tsp. roasted sesame seeds
- 1 tsp. salt

Directions:

1. Bring a medium-sized pot filled halfway with water to a boil over medium-high heat. Add the sugar snaps and cook them for about 2 minutes.

2. Take the pot off the heat, drain the excess water, transfer the sugar snaps to a medium-sized bowl, and set them aside for now.

3. Fill the pot with water again, add the teaspoon of salt and bring to a boil over medium-high heat. Add the edamame to the pot and let them cook for about 6 minutes.

4. Take the pot off the heat, drain the excess water, transfer the soybeans to the bowl with sugar snaps, and let them cool down for about 5 minutes.

5. Combine all ingredients, except the nori crumbs and roasted sesame seeds, in a medium-sized bowl. Carefully stir, using a spoon, until all ingredients are evenly coated in oil.

6. Top the salad with the nori crumbs and roasted sesame seeds. Transfer the bowl to the fridge and allow the salad to cool for at least 30 minutes. Serve chilled and enjoy!

Nutrition: Calories: 409 Carbs: 7.1 g. Fat: 38.25 g. Protein: 7.6 g.

14. __Flourless Bread__

Preparation time: 15 minutes

Cooking time: 40 minutes

Servings: 12

Ingredients:

- 1 tsp. coconut oil
- 6 tbsp. water
- 2 tbsp. flax seed (ground)
- 1 cup almond butter
- 1 cup pumpkin (pitted, diced, cooked. Alternatively, use canned pumpkin puree.)
- 1 ½ tsp baking powder
- ½ tsp cinnamon
- 1 cup of organic soy protein (vanilla flavor)
- ¼ cup pumpkin seeds (raw or roasted)
- Optional: ½ tsp. nutmeg

Directions:

1. Warm oven to 320°F/160°C. Prepare a large loaf pan lined using parchment paper and grease the paper with coconut oil.

2. In a small bowl, combine the water with the flax seeds. Allow the seeds to soak for about 10 minutes.

3. Put all the ingredients except the roasted pumpkin seeds in a blender or food processor. If desired, include the optional nutmeg.

4. Pulse until ingredients are combined into a smooth batter, scraping the blender or food processor's sides if necessary.

5. Move the batter into the loaf pan and allow the mixture to sit for a few minutes. Put the loaf pan in the oven and bake the bread for 20 minutes.

6. Remove the bread, then top it with the pumpkin seeds, then bake for another 15-20 minutes, or until a knife comes out clean. Remove the loaf pan out of the oven and allow the bread to cool.

7. Transfer the bread to a cutting board and slice it into 12 slices. Serve warm or cold and enjoy!

Nutrition: Calories: 191 Carbs: 3.3 g. Fat: 14.7 g. Protein: 10.8 g.

15. Walnut & Mushroom Loaf

Preparation time: 8 hours & 30 minutes

Cooking time: 60 minutes

Servings: 10

Ingredients:

- 2 tbsp. coconut oil
- 2 cups walnuts
- 3 portobello mushroom caps (stems removed)
- ½ cup green onion (sliced)
- 2 cups fresh baby spinach leaves

Marinade:

- 1 tbsp. balsamic vinegar
- 1 tbsp. soy sauce
- 1 tsp. cumin
- Pinch of Himalayan salt

Directions:

1. Grease a large cheese mold or loaf pan that fits in a dehydrator with coconut oil and set it aside.

2. In a medium-sized bowl, cover the walnuts with water and soak them for at least 8 hours. Rinse and drain the walnuts after soaking, and make sure no water is left.

3. Mix all the marinade fixings in a small bowl until no lumps remain. Cut the portobello mushroom caps into small pieces. Add to the marinade bowl and stir until all pieces are evenly coated. Set the mushrooms aside for 30 minutes.

4. After 30 minutes, put the walnuts into a food processor or blender and pulse into tiny bits. Add the marinated mushroom pieces and green onion and continue pulsing the ingredients into a smooth mixture with small chunks. It should take about 2 minutes.

5. Transfer the mixture into the cheese mold and sprinkle with some additional salt.

6. Cover the mold with parchment paper and place the walnut and mushroom loaf into a dehydrator. Dehydrate the loaf at 90°F/32°C for about 2 hours.

7. Flip the mold upside down and dehydrate for another 2 hours. Take the loaf out of the mold and cut it into 10 slices or chunks. Serve each slice with a handful of baby spinach leaves, and enjoy!

Nutrition: Calories: 195 Carbs: 2.9 g. Fat: 18.25 g. Protein: 4.5 g.

16. Tofu Stir-Fry Noodle Bowl

Preparation time: 15 minutes

Cooking time: 0 minutes

Servings: 2

Ingredients:

- 1 (12 oz. pack) extra firm tofu (drained, cubed)
- 2 (7 oz. packs) shirataki noodles
- 1 tbsp. coconut oil
- 1 tbsp. sesame oil
- 1 red bell pepper (seeded, chopped)
- 1 cup bok choi (finely chopped)

Sauce:

- 2 tbsp. Low-sodium soy sauce
- ½ tbsp. rice vinegar
- 1 tsp. chili garlic paste
- 1-inch piece ginger (finely chopped)
- 1 tsp. low-carb maple syrup
- 1 tsp. lemon juice
- 2 tsp. sesame oil

Toppings:

- ½ cup pickled red cabbage
- 1 medium Hass avocado (peeled, pitted, sliced)
- ¼ cup toasted sesame seeds

Directions:

1. In a medium-sized bowl, rinse the shirataki noodles with cold water, drain, and set aside.

2. Add the sauce ingredients to another medium-sized bowl and whisk thoroughly until smooth. Set the bowl aside—warm a large skillet over medium-high heat.

3. Add the coconut oil and sesame oil and stir until the skillet's bottom is coated and the oil is shimmering.

4. Add the tofu cubes and the chopped bell pepper to the skillet. Stir fry until the tofu cubes start to brown.

5. Add the bok choi, noodles, and sauce to the skillet and stir fry for another 5 minutes. Take the skillet off the heat and divide the tofu stir fry between two bowls.

6. Add some pickled red cabbage and avocado slices to each serving, garnish with sesame seeds, and enjoy!

Nutrition: Calories: 558 Carbs: 9.8 g. Fat: 46.65 g. Protein: 21.8 g.

17. Spicy Satay Tofu Salad

Preparation time: 15 minutes

Cooking time: 18 minutes

Servings: 2

Ingredients:

- 1 (12 oz. pack) extra-firm tofu (drained and cubed)
- ¼ cup peanut butter
- ½ tbsp. smoked paprika
- 1 tbsp sesame oil
- ¼ tbsp red chili flakes
- 2 drops liquid smoke
- 2 tbsp. water
- 1 tbsp. black sesame seeds

Salad:

- 4 cups fresh baby spinach leaves (rinsed, drained)
- ¼ cup fresh mint leaves (chopped)
- 2 tbsp. lemon juice
- 2 tbsp. avocado oil
- ¼ cup roasted cashews (unsalted)

Directions:

1. Warm oven to 400°F/200°C and lines a baking tray with parchment paper. Put the peanut butter, paprika, sesame oil, chili flakes, and liquid smoke into a large bowl.

2. Add the water to the bowl and mix thoroughly until all the ingredients are combined. Put the tofu cubes in the bowl with the peanut butter mixture and stir gently until all cubes are evenly covered.

3. Transfer the covered tofu cubes onto the baking tray, spread them out evenly, and sprinkle the sesame seeds over them.

4. Put the baking tray in your oven, then bake the tofu cubes for 18 minutes, or until browned and firm. Mix all the salad ingredients in a large bowl.

5. Take the tofu out of the oven and let the cubes cool for about 2 minutes. Divide the salad between two bowls, serve the tofu on top and enjoy!

Nutrition: Calories: 656.1 Carbs: 11.5 g. Fat: 54.4 g. Protein: 29 g.

18. Lemon Rosemary Almond Slices

Preparation time: 15 minutes

Cooking time: 20 minutes

Servings: 4

Ingredients:

- 1 (12 oz. pack) extra firm tofu (drained)
- 1 cup full-fat coconut milk
- 1 cup almond flour

Crust:

- ½ cup of raw almonds
- 1 sprig rosemary leaves (stems removed)
- 1 tbsp. organic lemon zest
- 1 tsp. Himalayan salt
- 1 garlic clove (minced)
- 1 tsp. ground black pepper

Directions:

1. Warm oven to 400°F/200°C and lines a baking tray using parchment paper. Press your tofu down on a plate to eliminate excess water and cut the block into 8 slices. Set the slices aside.

2. Put the almonds and rosemary into a food processor and process until chunky. Add the remaining crust fixings to the food processor and pulse until thoroughly combined.

3. Transfer mixture to a bowl. Pour the coconut milk into another medium-sized bowl and put the almond flour in a third medium-sized bowl.

4. Take a slice of tofu, dip each side in the bowl with almond flour and shake off any excess.

5. Dip the slice of flour-covered tofu into the coconut milk, and finally, dip it into the bowl with the lemon rosemary crust mix.

6. Place the coated slice of tofu onto the baking tray and repeat the process for all the tofu slices.

7. Put the tray in your oven, then bake the tofu slices for about 20 minutes, until browned and crispy.

8. Take the baking tray out of the oven and let the slices cool down for about a minute. Serve with a light salad of greens as a side dish and enjoy!

Nutrition: Calories: 442 Carbs: 5.2 g. Fat: 38.4 g. Protein: 17.9 g.

19. California Scramble Bowl

Preparation time: 15 minutes

Cooking time: 7 minutes

Servings: 2

Ingredients:

- 1 (10 oz. pack) extra firm smoked tofu (drained, scrambled)
- 2 tbsp. olive oil
- ½ green onion (finely chopped)
- 2 cloves garlic (minced)
- 1 jalapeño (seeded, finely chopped)
- 1 tsp dried oregano
- ½ tsp ground cumin
- ½ tsp smoked paprika

Salad:

- 4 cups iceberg lettuce (chopped)
- ¼ cup fresh cilantro (chopped)
- 1 large Hass avocado (peeled, pitted, sliced)
- 2 tbsp. lemon juice

Directions:

1. Put your large skillet over medium-high heat, then add the olive oil. Once the oil is warm and shimmering, add the onion and garlic. Stir fry until the ingredients start to caramelize.

2. Stir in the tofu scramble, chopped jalapeño, oregano, cumin, and smoked paprika. Stir-fry for about 7 minutes, then turn off the heat.

3. Divide the lettuce between two medium-sized bowls. Add half of the tofu scramble, chopped cilantro, and avocado slices to each. Top the avocado slices with lemon juice, serve and enjoy!

Nutrition: Calories: 428 Carbs: 9.3 g. Fat: 34.5 g. Protein: 18.2 g.

20. Steamed Eggplant with Cashew Dressing

Preparation time: 15 minutes

Cooking time: 0 minutes

Servings: 5

Ingredients:

- 3 small eggplants
- ¼ cup vegan mozzarella cheese
- 1 tbsp. water
- 1 tbsp. soy sauce
- 1 tbsp. chili oil
- 1 tbsp. toasted sesame seeds
- ½ shallot (minced)
- 1 tbsp. dried cilantro

Directions:

1. Fill a large pot (with a steamer on top) halfway with water and put it over medium-high heat. Halve the eggplants lengthwise and put them in the steamer basket once the water is simmering.

2. Steam the eggplant halves for about 15 minutes until they are soft and tender.

3. Meanwhile, add the vegan mozzarella, water, soy sauce, and chili oil to a medium-sized bowl and whisk thoroughly until all ingredients are combined.

4. Once the eggplant halves are cooked, remove them from the heat and arrange them on a medium platter.

5. Drizzle the mozzarella mixture over the eggplant halves and top with the sesame seeds, minced shallot, and cilantro. Serve warm and enjoy!

Nutrition: Calories: 168.5 Carbs: 9.8 g. Fat: 11.5 g. Protein: 4.9 g.

DINNER

21. Sushi Roll-Ups

Preparation Time: 20 minutes

Cooking Time: 0 minutes

Servings: 2

Ingredients:

For the dip/hummus:

- 1 fennel bulb
- A glug of olive oil
- 1 pinch of dried sage
- 1 tbsp. tahini
- A handful of almonds
- 3 ½ oz chickpeas from a can, drained
- Pinch salt
- Juice of ½ lemon

For the Roll-Ups:

- 1 capsicum sliced into matchsticks
- 1 small bunch of cilantros
- 1 avocado, sliced

- 1 cucumber, cut into matchsticks

- 1 parsnip, cut into matchsticks

- 2 medium zucchinis

Directions:

1. Pulse all the Ingredients for the hummus in a blender. Add a bit of lemon and olive oil to get your desired consistency.

2. To make the roll-ups, first, chop the zucchini into long thin strips. Then lay individual zucchini strips out and spread a generous amount of almond hummus onto the zucchini strip.

3. Now add little amounts of the avocado, cucumber, and the matchsticks of veggies. Top with some sesame seeds, and then serve.

Nutrition: Calories: 743 Fat: 51g Carb: 50g Protein: 31g

22. Mushroom "Chicken Tenders"

Preparation Time: 1 hour

Cooking Time: 30 minutes

Servings: 6

Ingredients:

- Grapeseed oil as needed
- 1 tsp. ground cloves
- 1 tsp. cayenne powder
- 2 tsp. ginger powder
- 2 tsp. onion powder
- 2 tsp. sage
- 2 tsp sea salt
- 2 tsp. basil
- 2 tsp. oregano
- 1 ½ cup spelt flour
- 1 ½ cups spring flour
- 2 to 6 Portobello mushrooms

Directions:

1. Slice the mushrooms caps approximately half-inch apart. Add mushrooms, oil, water, and half of the individual seasonings to the bowl and mix for 1 hour.

2. In a separate bowl, blend the rest of the seasonings and the spelt flour and then batter the mushrooms.

3. Preheat oven to 400F. Grease a baking sheet with grapeseed oil and put the mushrooms on the baking sheet. Bake 15 minutes per side, or until crispy. Serve.

Nutrition: Calories: 276 Fat: 6.5g Carb: 49.48g Protein: 10.72g

23. Quinoa Pasta with Tomato Artichoke Sauce

Preparation Time: 10 minutes

Cooking Time: 20 minutes

Servings: 2

Ingredients:

- 2 tbsp extra-virgin olive oil
- 1 pinch cayenne pepper
- ½ tsp. sea salt
- 3 tbsp. basil, fresh
- 1 tsp. vegetable stock
- 1-ounce walnuts
- 1 fennel bulb
- 1 onion, chopped
- 8 ounces artichoke hearts
- 5 ounces cherry tomatoes, fresh
- 7 ounces quinoa or spelt pasta

Directions:

1. Cook the artichoke until tender. Then cook the pasta as stated in the package Directions. Chopped all the veggies.

2. Heat 2 tablespoons of oil and stir fry onions, nuts, and fennel for a few minutes. Then add the cooked artichokes and tomatoes and cook for 2 minutes.

3. Scoop about ½ cup of water and then dissolve the vegetable stock into the water. Add into a pan and simmer for 2 minutes on low heat. Stir regularly. Add basil, season with salt and pepper. Put the sauce on the pasta and serve.

Nutrition: Calories: 719 Fat: 26g Carb: 111g Protein: 23.9g

24. Alkalizing Tahini Noodle Bowl

Preparation Time: 10 minutes

Cooking Time: 0 minutes

Servings: 2

Ingredients:

- 1 tsp. black sesame seeds
- ½ avocado, chopped
- 2 green onions, chopped
- 4 kale, chopped
- 1 parsnip, shredded
- 4 leaves of romaine, chopped
- 1 yellow zucchini, spiralized
- Dressing:
- 1 tsp. agave
- 2 tbsp. lemon juice
- 1 tbsp. tahini
- Dash of salt

Directions:

1. Put all the vegetables you chopped in a bowl. Add all Ingredients for dressing in another bowl and whisk.

Pour the dressing over the vegetables and garnish with sesame seeds.

Nutrition: Calories: 209 Fat: 14.5g Carb: 22.07g Protein: 5.49g

25. Alkaline Meatloaf

Preparation Time: 15 minutes

Cooking Time: 70 minutes

Servings: 1 loaf

Ingredients:

- 1 cup prepared wild rice
- ½ cup homemade tomato sauce, divided
- ½ cup chopped yellow onion, divided
- ½ cup chopped green bell pepper, divided
- 1 shallot, chopped
- 2 cups mixed mushrooms, chopped
- ¼ tsp. cloves
- ½ tsp. ginger
- ½ tsp. tarragon
- 1 tsp. thyme
- 1 tsp. sage
- 1 tbsp. sea salt
- 1 tbsp. onion powder
- 1 cup garbanzo flour or spelt flour
- cups breadcrumbs (made of spelt flour)
- 2 cups cooked chickpeas

- Cayenne to taste

Directions:

1. Clean and dry wild rice. Prepare the chickpeas as well and set them aside. Mix garbanzo flour or spelt flour with bread crumbs and set the mixture aside.

2. Chop the green peppers and the onions and place half of each of them to the side.

3. Now chop the shallots and mushrooms and add them to a food processor, along with chickpeas, half of the onion, half of the green peppers, and spices.

4. Pulse the mixture until fully incorporated. Then add in 2 tbsp of tomato sauce and the wild rice. And continue to blend until a paste.

5. Move the mixture to a mixing bowl. Add the remaining flour, bread crumbs, onion, and green pepper. Mix well.

6. Pour the mixture into a greased pan and cover with the remaining tomato sauce—Bake in the preheated oven at 350F within 60 to 70 minutes. Cool, slice, and serve.

Nutrition: Calories: 265 Fat: 2.96g Carb: 48g Protein: 13.15g

26. Pizza

Preparation Time: 15 minutes

Cooking Time: 30 minutes

Servings: 6

Ingredients:

For the crust:

- 1 ½ cups spelt flour
- 1 cup spring water
- ½ tsp onion powder
- ½ tsp oregano
- ½ tsp sea salt
- ½ tsp basil

Cheese:

- ¼ tsp sea salt
- ½ tsp basil
- ½ tsp oregano
- ½ tsp. onion powder
- 1 tsp. lime juice
- ¼ cup hemp milk/nut milk
- ½ cup spring water

- 1 cup Brazil nuts, soaked overnight

Toppings:

- Homemade tomato sauce as needed
- 3 tbsp. red onion chopped
- ½ plum tomato, sliced

Directions:

1. Combine all the seasonings in a bowl with spelt flour and then add in half a water cup. Add more water if needed.
2. Make a dough and roll on a floured surface, then place the dough into a baking sheet that is gently coated with oil. Poke holes with a fork.
3. Bake within 10 to 15 minutes in the preheated oven at 350F. Meanwhile, add all Ingredients for cheese in a blender and process until smooth.
4. Once the crust is cooked, coat it with the cheese, sauce, and toppings. Bake again in the bottom rack at 425F for 10 to 15 minutes more. Enjoy.

Nutrition: Calories: 322 Fat: 18g Carb: 34g Protein: 9g

27. **Alkaline Electric Veggie Lasagna**

Preparation Time: 1 hour

Cooking Time: 70 minutes

Servings: 6

Ingredients:

Pasta:

- Spelt lasagna sheets as needed

Meat alternative:

- 1 tsp. fennel powder
- 2 tsp. basil
- 2 tsp. oregano
- 1 tbsp. sea salt
- 2 tbsp. onion powder
- ½ cup tomato sauce
- 1 cup red peppers, diced
- 1 cup onions, chopped
- 1 cup cooked chickpeas/garbanzo beans
- 2 cups cooked spelt berries/kernels
- Brazil Nut Cheese
- 1 tsp. basil

- 1 tsp. oregano
- 1 tsp. sea salt
- 1 tbsp. onion powder
- 1 tbsp. hemp seeds
- 1 cup spring water
- 2 cups-soaked Brazil nuts

Extras:

- White mushrooms
- Grapeseed oil as needed
- Zucchini as needed

Directions:

1. Combine all the meat alternatives in a food processor and blend until mixed. Grease a skillet using grapeseed oil and heat over medium heat. Sauté peppers and onions for 5 minutes.

2. Add the garbanzo and spelt mixture from the food processor. Put some grapeseed oil in the skillet and cook the mixture for 10 to 12 minutes.

3. In a blender, add the cheese Ingredients and 1 cup of water and process until smooth. Reserve a cup of

tomato sauce and then pour the rest of the sauce into the garbanzo bean and spelt mixture. Mix.

4. Slice the zucchini and mushrooms lengthwise. Coat the bottom of the dish using the reserved tomato sauce.

5. Then lay the spelt pasta, sliced zucchini, the garbanzo/spelt mixture, alkaline cheese, white mushrooms, and spelt pasta again.

6. Repeat until you get 4 layers of the pasta. Then top the last layer with the garbanzo/spelt mixture and cheese.

7. Pour the rest of the tomato sauce around the lasagna layers and sprinkle with some dried basil. Bake at 350F for 35 to 45 minutes. Cool and serve.

Nutrition: Calories: 575 Fat: 36g Carb: 60g Protein: 11.5g

28. Zucchini Pasta

Preparation Time: 10 minutes

Cooking Time: 5 minutes

Servings: 2

Ingredients:

- 4 zucchinis, large and spiralized
- ¼ tsp. salt
- 2 avocados, chopped
- 2 tbsp. grapeseed oil
- 1 cup cherry tomatoes
- ¼ cup basil, fresh

Directions:

1. Warm-up the oil in a skillet, cook the zoodles for 5 minutes and then transfer to a large bowl. Stir in the cherry tomatoes, avocado, salt, and basil. Mix and serve.

Nutrition: Calories: 610 Fat: 53.7g Carb: 34g Protein: 9.4g

29. Egg Foo Yung

Preparation Time: 10 minutes

Cooking Time: 15 minutes

Servings: 6

Ingredients:

- Grapeseed oil as needed
- 1 cup spring water
- 1/8 tsp. ginger powder
- ½ tsp. cayenne powder
- 1 tsp. oregano
- 1 tsp. sea salt
- 1 tsp. onion powder
- 1 tsp. basil
- ¾ cup garbanzo bean flour
- ½ cup red and white onion, chopped
- ½ cup green onions, chopped
- ½ cup red and green peppers, chopped
- 1 cup butternut squash, chopped
- 2 cups mushrooms, sliced
- 3 cups prepared spaghetti squash

Directions:

1. In a bowl, whisk the garbanzo flour, seasonings, and spring water. Then add the veggies and prepared spaghetti squash. Combine to mix.

2. Coat a skillet with grapeseed oil and add ½ cup of the mixture to the pan. Pat down the dough into patties and cook 3 to 4 minutes on each side. Serve.

Nutrition: Calories: 139 Fat: 2.1g Carb: 24.7g Protein: 6.6g

30. Lentil & Chickpeas Salad

Preparation time: 15 minutes

Cooking time: 35 minutes

Servings: 6

Ingredients:

Lentils:

- 4 cups water
- 2 cups dried green lentils, rinsed
- 2 large garlic cloves, halved lengthwise
- 2 tablespoons olive oil

Dressing:

- 1 garlic clove, minced
- ¼ cup fresh lemon juice
- 2 tablespoons olive oil
- 1 teaspoon maple syrup
- 1 teaspoon Dijon mustard
- Salt and ground black pepper, to taste

Salad:

- 1½ (15-ounce) cans chickpeas, rinsed and drained
- 2 large avocados, peeled, pitted, and chopped

- 2 cups radishes, trimmed and sliced
- ¼ cup fresh mint leaves, chopped

Directions:

1. For lentil, add all ingredients in a medium pot over medium-high heat and bring to a boil.
2. Then, adjust the heat to low and simmer for about 25–35 minutes or until the lentils are cooked through and tender. Drain the lentils and discard the garlic cloves.
3. For dressing, add all ingredients in a small bowl and beat until well combined. In a large serving bowl, add lentils, chickpeas, radishes, avocados, and mint, and mix. Add dressing and toss to coat well. Serve immediately.

Nutrition: Calories 561 Fat 22.2 g Carbs 66.4 g Protein 24.9 g

SNACKS

31. Chipotle and Lime Tortilla Chips

Preparation time: 10 minutes

Cooking time: 15 minutes

Servings: 4

Ingredients:

- 12 ounces whole-wheat tortillas
- 4 tablespoons chipotle seasoning
- 1 tablespoon olive oil
- 4 limes, juiced

Directions:

1. Whisk together oil and lime juice, brush it well on tortillas, then sprinkle with chipotle seasoning and bake for 15 minutes at 350 degrees F until crispy, turning halfway.
2. When done, let the tortilla cool for 10 minutes, then break it into chips and serve.

Nutrition: Calories: 150 Fat: 7 g Carbs: 18 g Protein: 2 g

32. Carrot and Sweet Potato Fritters

Preparation time: 10 minutes

Cooking time: 8 minutes

Servings: 10

Ingredients:

- 1/3 cup quinoa flour

- 1½ cups shredded sweet potato

- 1 cup grated carrot

- 1/3 teaspoon ground black pepper

- 2/3 teaspoon salt

- 2 teaspoons curry powder

- 2 flax eggs

- 2 tablespoons coconut oil

Directions:

1. Place all the fixings in a bowl, except for oil, stir well until combined and then shape the mixture into ten small patties

2. Take a large pan, place it over medium-high heat, add oil and when it melts, add patties in it and cook for 3 minutes per side until browned. Serve straight away

Nutrition: Calories: 70 Fat: 3 g Carbs: 8 g Protein: 1 g

33. Buffalo Quinoa Bites

Preparation time: 15 minutes

Cooking time: 30 minutes

Servings: 20

Ingredients:

For the Bites:

- 1 cup cooked quinoa
- 15 ounces cooked white beans
- 3 tablespoons chickpea flour
- 1 medium shallot, peeled, chopped
- 3 cloves of garlic, peeled
- ½ teaspoon ground black pepper
- 1/2 teaspoon salt
- 1 teaspoon smoked paprika
- 1/4 cup vegan buffalo sauce

For the Dressing:

- 1/4 cup chives
- 2 tablespoons hemp hearts
- 1 tablespoon nutritional yeast
- 1 teaspoon garlic powder

- 1 teaspoon onion powder
- 1/2 teaspoon salt
- ½ teaspoon ground black pepper
- 2 teaspoons dried dill
- 1 lemon, juiced
- 1/4 cup tahini
- 3/4 cup water

Directions:

1. Prepare the bites, and for this, place half of the beans in a food processor, add garlic and shallots, and pulse for 2 minutes until mixture comes together.
2. Then add all the spices of the bites and buffalo sauce and pulse for 2 minutes until smooth. Add remaining beans along with chickpea flour and quinoa and pulse until just combined.
3. Tip the mixture in a dish, shape it in the dough, shape it into twenty balls, about the golf-ball size, and bake for 30 minutes at 350 degrees F until crispy and browned, turning halfway.
4. Meanwhile, prepare the dressing and for this, place all of its ingredients in a food processor and pulse for 2

minutes until smooth. Serve bites with prepared dressing.

Nutrition: Calories: 78 Fat: 3 g Carbs: 9 g Protein: 4 g

34. <u>Tomato and Pesto Toast</u>

Preparation time: 5 minutes

Cooking time: 0 minute

Servings: 4

Ingredients:

- 1 small tomato, sliced
- ¼ teaspoon ground black pepper
- 1 tablespoon vegan pesto
- 2 tablespoons hummus
- 1 slice of whole-grain bread, toasted
- Hemp seeds as needed for garnishing

Directions:

1. Spread hummus on one side of the toast, top with tomato slices and then drizzle with pesto.
2. Sprinkle black pepper on the toast along with hemp seeds and then serve straight away.

Nutrition: Calories: 214 Fat: 7.2 g Carbs: 32 g Protein: 6.5 g

35. Avocado and Sprout Toast

Preparation time: 5 minutes

Cooking time: 0 minute

Servings: 4

Ingredients:

- 1/2 of a medium avocado, sliced
- 1 slice of whole-grain bread, toasted
- 2 tablespoons sprouts
- 2 tablespoons hummus
- ¼ teaspoon lemon zest
- ½ teaspoon hemp seeds
- ¼ teaspoon red pepper flakes

Directions:

1. Spread hummus on one side of the toast and then top with avocado slices and sprouts. Sprinkle with lemon zest, hemp seeds, and red pepper flakes and then serve straight away.

Nutrition: Calories: 200 Fat: 10.5 g Carbs: 22 g Protein: 7 g

36. Apple and Honey Toast

Preparation time: 5 minutes

Cooking time: 0 minute

Servings: 4

Ingredients:

- ½ of a small apple, cored, sliced
- 1 slice of whole-grain bread, toasted
- 1 tablespoon honey
- 2 tablespoons hummus
- 1/8 teaspoon cinnamon

Directions:

1. Spread hummus on one side of the toast, top with apple slices and then drizzle with honey.
2. Sprinkle cinnamon on it and then serve straight away.

Nutrition: Calories: 212 Fat: 7 g Carbs: 35 g Protein: 4 g

37. Thai Snack Mix

Preparation time: 15 minutes

Cooking time: 90 minutes

Servings: 4

Ingredients:

- 5 cups mixed nuts
- 1 cup chopped dried pineapple
- 1 cup pumpkin seed
- 1 teaspoon onion powder
- 1 teaspoon garlic powder
- 2 teaspoons paprika
- 1/2 teaspoon ground black pepper
- 1 teaspoon of sea salt
- 1/4 cup coconut sugar
- 1/2 teaspoon red chili powder
- 1 tablespoon red pepper flakes
- 1/2 tablespoon red curry powder
- 2 tablespoons soy sauce
- 2 tablespoons coconut oil

Directions:

1. Switch on the slow cooker, add all the ingredients in it except for dried pineapple and red pepper flakes, stir until combined and cook for 90 minutes at high heat setting, stirring every 30 minutes.

2. When done, spread the nut mixture on a baking sheet lined with parchment paper and let it cool. Then spread dried pineapple on top, sprinkle with red pepper flakes and serve.

Nutrition: Calories: 230 Fat: 17.5 g Carbs: 11.5 g Protein: 6.5 g

38. Zucchini Fritters

Preparation time: 10 minutes

Cooking time: 6 minutes

Servings: 12

Ingredients:

- 1/2 cup quinoa flour
- 3 1/2 cups shredded zucchini
- 1/2 cup chopped scallions
- 1/3 teaspoon ground black pepper
- 1 teaspoon salt
- 2 tablespoons coconut oil
- 2 flax eggs

Directions:

1. Squeeze moisture from the zucchini by wrapping it in a cheesecloth and then transfer it to a bowl. Add remaining ingredients, except for oil, stir until combined and then shape the mixture into twelve patties.

2. Take a skillet pan, place it over medium-high heat, add oil and when hot, add patties and cook for 3 minutes

per side until brown. Serve the patties with favorite vegan sauce.

Nutrition: Calories: 37 Fat: 1 g Carbs: 4 g Protein: 2 g

39. Zucchini Chips

Preparation time: 10 minutes

Cooking time: 120 minutes

Servings: 4

Ingredients:

- 1 large zucchini, thinly sliced
- 1 teaspoon salt
- 2 tablespoons olive oil

Directions:

1. Pat dry zucchini slices and then spread them in an even layer on a baking sheet lined with parchment sheet.

2. Whisk together salt and oil, brush this mixture over zucchini slices on both sides and then bake for 2 hours or more until brown and crispy. When done, let the chips cool for 10 minutes and then serve straight away.

Nutrition: Calories: 54 Fat: 5 g Carbs: 1 g Protein: 0 g

40. Rosemary Beet Chips

Preparation time: 10 minutes

Cooking time: 20 minutes

Servings: 3

Ingredients:

- 3 large beets, scrubbed, thinly sliced
- 1/8 teaspoon ground black pepper
- ¼ teaspoon of sea salt
- 3 sprigs of rosemary, leaves chopped
- 4 tablespoons olive oil

Directions:

1. Spread beet slices in a single layer between two large baking sheets, brush the slices with oil, then season with spices and rosemary, toss until well coated, and bake for 20 minutes at 375 degrees F until crispy, turning halfway.

2. When done, let the chips cool for 10 minutes and then serve.

Nutrition: Calories: 79 Fat: 4.7 g Carbs: 8.6 g Protein: 1.5 g

DESSERT RECIPES

41. Everyday Energy Bars

Preparation time: 15 minutes

Cooking time: 33 minutes

Servings: 16

Ingredients:

- 1 cup vegan butter
- 1 cup brown sugar
- 2 tablespoons agave syrup
- 2 cups old-fashioned oats
- 1/2 cup almonds, slivered
- 1/2 cup walnuts, chopped
- 1/2 cup dried currants
- 1/2 cup pepitas

Directions:

1. Warm your oven to 320 degrees F. Line a baking pan with parchment paper or Silpat mat. Thoroughly combine all the ingredients until everything is well incorporated.

2. Spread the mixture onto the prepared baking pan using a wide spatula. Bake for about 33 minutes or until golden brown. Slice into bars using a sharp knife and enjoy!

Nutrition: Calories: 285 Fat: 17.1g Carbs: 30g Protein: 5.1g

42. <u>Chocolate Hazelnut Fudge</u>

Preparation time: 1 hour & 15 minutes

Cooking time: 0 minutes

Servings: 20

Ingredients:

- 1 cup cashew butter
- 1 cup fresh dates, pitted
- 1/4 cup cocoa powder
- 1/4 teaspoon ground cloves
- 1 teaspoon matcha powder
- 1 teaspoon vanilla extract
- 1/2 cup hazelnuts, coarsely chopped

Directions:

1. Process all ingredients in your blender until uniform and smooth. Scrape the batter into a parchment-lined baking sheet. Place it in your freezer for at least 1 hour to set. Cut into squares and serve. Bon appétit!

Nutrition: Calories: 127 Fat: 9g Carbs: 10.7g Protein: 2.4g

43. No-Bake Pumpkin Pie

Preparation Time: 10 minutes

Cooking Time: 0 minutes

Servings: 8

Ingredients:

- 1 cup pumpkin puree
- 2 tsp pumpkin pie spice
- oz. vanilla pudding
- 8-ounce cool whip
- ¼ cup milk
- 1 graham cracker crust
- Whipped cream for garnish

Directions:

1. Take a bowl pour pumpkin puree in it, add pudding mix, pumpkin pie spice and milk. Mix the Ingredients well until they turn smooth.

2. Now fold it into cool whip carefully. Take a graham cracker in a pie pan and spread the pumpkin puree on the pie and spread well. Chill it well before serving, and serve with whipped cream topping.

Nutrition Calories: 323 Carbs: 42g Fat: 15g Protein: 6g

44. Vegan Vanilla Almond Cookies

Preparation Time: 15 minutes

Cooking Time: 45 minutes

Servings: 10

Ingredients:

- 2 cups all-purpose flour
- 1 cup almond meal
- ½ tsp. salt
- 1 cup powdered sugar
- 1 cup vegan butter
- ½ tsp. almond extract
- 2 tsp. vanilla
- 20 almonds

Directions:

1. Warm your oven to 350 degrees Fahrenheit. Mix your dry fixings in a large bowl. Put the wet fixings, and stir well to create a dough. Don't add the almonds.
2. Next, roll your dough into a log with a two-inch diameter, and slice the cookie roll into flat cookies—like you would slice a cucumber.

3. Put the cookies on your baking sheet, and press the almonds into the cookies. Bake the cookies within 20 minutes in the preheated oven, and enjoy.

Nutrition Calories: 180 Carbs: 13g Fat: 14g Protein: 4g

45. <u>Onion Cheese Muffins</u>

Preparation Time: 20 minutes

Cooking Time: 20 minutes

Servings: 6

Ingredients:

- ¼ cup Colby jack cheese, shredded
- ¼ cup shallots, minced
- 1 cup almond flour
- 1 organic egg
- 3 tbsp sour cream
- ½ tsp salt
- 3 tbsp melted butter or oil

Directions:

1. Line 6 muffin tins with 6 muffin liners. Set aside and preheat oven to 350F. In a bowl, stir the dry and wet ingredients alternately. Mix well using a spatula until the consistency of the mixture becomes even.

2. Scoop a spoonful of the batter to the prepared muffin tins. Bake for 20 minutes in the oven until golden brown. Serve and enjoy.

Nutrition: Calories: 153 Carbs: 27g Fat: 3g Protein: 5g

46. **French Lover's Coconut Macaroons**

Preparation Time: 15 minutes

Cooking Time: 25 minutes

Servings: 6

Ingredients:

- 1/3 cup agave nectar
- ½ cup coconut cream
- 1 cup shredded coconut
- ½ tsp. salt
- 1/3 cup chocolate chips

Directions:

1. Warm your oven to 300 degrees Fahrenheit. Mix the coconut cream, the agave, and the salt. Fold in the chocolate chips plus the coconut.
2. Stir well, and create cookie balls. Place the balls on a baking sheet, and bake the cookies for twenty-five minutes. Enjoy.

Nutrition Calories: 57 Carbs: 3g Fat: 4g Protein: 3g

47. Oatmeal Raisin Cookies

Preparation Time: 15 minutes

Cooking Time: 35 minutes

Servings: 12

Ingredients:

- 1 cup whole wheat flour
- ½ tsp. salt
- ½ tsp. baking soda
- 1 tsp. cinnamon
- ½ cup brown sugar
- 2 tbsp. maple syrup
- ½ cup sugar
- 1/3 cup applesauce
- ½ tsp. vanilla
- 1/3 cup olive oil
- ½ cup raisins
- 1 ¾ cup oats

Directions:

1. Warm the oven to 350 degrees Fahrenheit. Next, mix together all the dry ingredients. Place this mixture to the side.

2. Mix all the wet fixings in a large mixing bowl. Put the dry fixings to the wet fixings slowly, stirring as you go. Add the oats next, stirring well. Lastly, add the raisins.

3. Let your batter to chill in the fridge within twenty minutes. Afterwards, drop the cookies onto a baking sheet and bake them for thirteen minutes. Enjoy after cooling.

Nutrition: Calories: 145 Carbs: 22g Fat: 5g Protein: 2g

48. Zucchini Chocolate Crisis Bread

Preparation Time: 15 minutes

Cooking Time: 25 minutes

Servings: 8

Ingredients:

- 1 cup sugar
- 2 tbsp. flax seeds
- 6 tbsp. water
- 1 cup applesauce
- 1/3 cup cocoa powder
- 2 cups all-purpose flour
- 2 tsp. vanilla
- 1 tsp. baking soda
- ½ tsp. baking powder
- 1 tbsp. cinnamon
- 1 tsp. salt
- 2 1/3 cup grated zucchini
- 1 cup nondairy chocolate chips

Directions:

1. Warm your oven to 325 degrees Fahrenheit. First, mix together the water and the flax seeds and allow the mixture to thicken to the side for five minutes.

2. Mix all the dry ingredients together. Next, add the wet ingredients to the dry ingredients, including the flax seeds. Next, add the chocolate chips and the zucchini.

3. Stir well, and spread the batter out into your bread loaf pan. Bake the creation for thirty minutes. Afterward it cools, enjoy!

Nutrition: Calories: 110 Carbs: 16g Fat: 5g Protein: 2g

49. Banana Blueberry Bread

Preparation Time: 15 minutes

Cooking Time: 35 minutes

Servings: 8

Ingredients:

- 3 tbsp. lemon juice
- 4 bananas
- ½ cup agave nectar
- ½ cup vegan milk
- 1 ¾ cup all-purpose flour
- 1 tsp. baking soda
- 1 tsp. baking powder
- 1 tsp. salt
- 2 cups blueberries

Directions:

1. Warm your oven to 350 degrees Fahrenheit. Mix the dry fixings in a large bowl and your wet ingredients in a different, smaller bowl. Make sure to mash up the bananas well.

2. Stir the ingredients together in the large bowl, making sure to assimilate the ingredients together completely.

3. Add the blueberries last, and then pour the mixture into a bread pan. Allow the bread to bake for fifty minutes, and enjoy.

Nutrition: Calories: 155 Carbs: 31g Fat: 2g Protein: 5g

50. Apple Cobbler Pie

Preparation Time: 15 minutes

Cooking Time: 25 minutes

Servings: 3

Ingredients:

- 3 cups sliced apples
- 6 cups sliced peaches
- 2 tbsp. arrowroot powder
- ½ cup white sugar
- 1 tsp. cinnamon
- 1 tsp. vanilla
- ½ cup water

Biscuit Topping Ingredients:

- ½ cup almond flour
- 1 cup gluten-free ground-up oats
- ½ tsp. salt
- 2 tsp. baking powder
- 2 tbsp. white sugar
- 1 tsp. cinnamon
- ½ cup soymilk
- 4 tbsp. vegan butter

Directions:

1. Warm your oven to 400 degrees Fahrenheit. Next, coat the peaches and the apples with the sugar, arrowroot, the cinnamon, the vanilla, and the water in a large bowl.

2. Allow the mixture to boil in a saucepan. After it begins to boil, allow the apples and peaches to simmer for three minutes. Remove the fruit from the heat and add the vanilla.

3. Now, add the dry ingredients together in a small bowl. Cut the biscuit with the vegan butter to create a crumble. Add the almond milk, and cover the fruit with this batter.

4. Bake this mixture for thirty minutes. Serve warm, and enjoy!

Nutrition: Calories: 270 Carbs: 39g Fat: 12g Protein: 2g

CONCLUSION

A plant based diet is a way of eating that is characterized by a heavy focus on fruits, vegetables, and whole grains, with few or no animal-based products.

A plant-based diet helps to prevent or manage many diseases including heart disease, cancer and type 2 diabetes.

The USDA recommends that at least ¼ of your plate (or a minimum of 600 calories) consist of fruit and vegetables to ensure you're getting the vitamins and minerals you need to stay healthy; this is specifically important for people with chronic health conditions like high blood pressure, high cholesterol or type 2 diabetes.

A plant-based diet is a great option for people who want to reduce their intake of saturated fat while maintaining or increasing their intake of fiber, vitamins and other nutrients. A plant-based diet can also reduce the risk of developing heart disease, type 2 diabetes, stroke and certain types of cancer.

In terms of weight loss, research have shown that a plant-based diet can help you lose weight if that's your goal.

A plant-based diet has many other health benefits as well.

The nutrient profile of a plant-based diet is similar to that of the Mediterranean Diet, which is often used as a model for dieting and eating healthy. However, the main difference is that a Mediterranean diet usually contains plenty of fatty fish (like salmon) along with nuts, cheese, high-fat dairy products and sometimes lamb.

While fish provides essential fatty acids like DHA, EPA and Omega 3s these can be difficult to obtain through food sources alone in modern diets.

One study showed that people who follow a plant-based diet are about 10 pounds lighter than meat eaters in their 30s and 40s. The research study also found that about one third of participants lost 10 percent or more of their body weight within two years.

As a vegan, you're sure to experience the benefits of a plant-based diet. But, how exactly can it help with weight loss? Or how about controlling blood sugar and cholesterol?

Dietary Guidelines: The official documents released by government authorities that explain our food recommendations for healthy living. These recommendations were formed using scientific research and advice from health experts across North America.